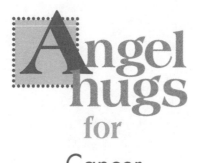

Angel hugs for

Cancer Patients

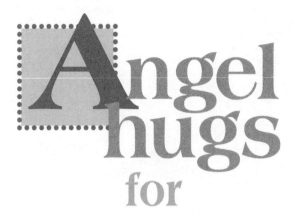

Angel hugs for

Cancer
Patients

LaDonna Meinders

CHALICE
PRESS

ST. LOUIS, MISSOURI

All Bible quotations, unless otherwise noted, are from the *Revised Standard Version of the Bible*, copyright 1952, [2nd edition, 1971] by the Division of Christian Education of the National Council of the Churches of Christ in the United States of America. Used by permission. All rights reserved.

Scripture quotations marked (NIV) are taken from the HOLY BIBLE, NEW INTERNATIONAL VERSION®. NIV®. Copyright © 1973, 1978, 1984 by International Bible Society. Used by permission of Zondervan Publishing House. All rights reserved.

Scripture quotations marked NKJV are taken from the *New King James Version*. Copyright © 1979, 1980, 1982 by Thomas Nelson, Inc. Used by permission. All rights reserved.

Scripture quotations marked (TLB) are taken from *The Living Bible*, copyright © 1971. Used by permission of Tyndale House Publishers, Inc., Wheaton, Illinois 60189. All rights reserved.

Scripture quotations marked (NLT) are taken from the Holy Bible, *New Living Translation*, copyright © 1996. Used by permission of Tyndale House Publishers, Inc., Wheaton, Illinois 60189, U.S.A. All rights reserved.

Cover art: Chris Sharp
Cover and interior design: Elizabeth Wright
Art direction: Elizabeth Wright

This book is printed on acid-free, recycled paper.

Visit Chalice Press on the World Wide Web at
www.chalicepress.com

10 9 8 7 6 5 4 3 2 1   04   05   06   07   08   09

Library of Congress Cataloging-in-Publication Data

Meinders, LaDonna Kramer.
 Angel hugs for cancer patients/LaDonna Meinders.
    p. cm.
ISBN 0-8272-0028-5
1. Cancer--Patients--Religious life. I. Title.
BV4910.33.M45 2004
242'.4--dc22

                                                              2003026294

Printed in the United States of America

Contents

●●●●●●●●●●●●●●●●●●●●●●●●●●●●●●●●

Foreword

●●●●●●●●●●●●●●●●●●●●●●●●●●●●●●●●●●●●●

Good morning, Americans! You are holding in your hands a book that will make a positive difference in your life every day *for the next thirty-one days… and, I predict, long afterward.*

In my career as a radio commentator, writer, and public speaker, I cannot overstate the importance of words. Words are powerful tools that can build confidence, convince, encourage, and yes, even heal. The words in LaDonna Meinders' book are jam-packed with inspiration and unforgettable stories that will touch your heart.

Cancer is epidemic in our great country. We are now told that one in three of us will get cancer. None of us ever want to hear those words, "You have cancer," and yet you and I rub elbows every day with courageous men and women who have heard those words and overcome them. They are cancer survivors! Now, most of the time, you will never know this, because these people have a spring in their step and a sparkle in their eyes. They are role models for all of us.

For those of you undergoing treatment, this book can be a medicine as potent as that bottle of pills you open every morning, because we now know that courage, hope, and a sense of humor are some of the best prescriptions for getting well!

Cancer never leaves us the way it finds us. And yes, my friends, sometimes it leaves us better *than before! I say better because it can leave us with a new appreciation for loved ones and for life itself. When you've read the stories in this book, you'll see what I mean.*

Share this book with someone who is hurting. You will both be blessed.

Paul Harvey

Acknowledgments

There are many people who helped bring this book to life. Their collective "Angel Hug" has been a blessing to me and will, I trust, bring hope and cheer to readers whose lives have been interrupted by cancer.

To Paul Harvey, whom I consider a true "voice of America," I owe a huge debt of thanks for your delightful Foreword.

I am grateful to those whose endorsements appear on the book jacket. Thank you, Governor George Nigh, Dr. William Tabbernee, Robert Funk, Barbara Green, and Dean Marvel Williamson. Your encouragement and endorsement of my work are a great honor to me.

To Mo Grotjohn, a friend and proofreader of the first order, and to Evelyn Chappell, my heartfelt thanks. You both always took time from your busy schedules to offer help when it was needed.

To those dear friends who allowed me to interview them and share the stories of their battles with cancer: Words are inadequate to tell you how much I appreciate and admire you! Your willingness to tell your personal stories of cancer will touch every reader and give more hope and courage than you will ever know. Thank you from the bottom of my heart!

As always, my family was supportive and encouraging as the book progressed. To my husband Herman and all the rest of you whom I am privileged to call my family, my deepest thanks. A special hug is due you if I wrote about you in the book.

I end with a prayer for those of you facing cancer today, or those whose loved one is doing so. May you feel God's healing presence and know that you are not alone.

LaDonna Meinders

Cancer is so limited…

*It cannot cripple **Love***
    *It cannot shatter **Hope***
        *It cannot erode **Faith***
            *It cannot destroy **Peace***

*It cannot wipe out **Confidence***
    *It cannot kill **Friendship***
        *It cannot suppress **Memories***
            *It cannot silence **Courage***

*It cannot invade the **Soul***
    *It cannot steal **Eternal Life***
        *It cannot conquer the **Spirit***
            *It cannot lessen the power of **Resurrection***

SEEN IN PHYSICIAN'S OFFICE, AUTHOR UNKNOWN

Green Pastures

• •

The LORD is my shepherd, I shall not want;
he makes me lie down in green pastures.
He leads me beside still waters;
he restores my soul.
He leads me in paths of righteousness
for his name's sake.
Even though I walk through the valley of the shadow
of death,
I fear no evil;
for thou art with me;
thy rod and thy staff,
they comfort me.

PSALMS 23:1–4

It was merely an enlarged lymph node discovered in a routine examination. When the doctor suggested a biopsy, I wasn't worried. I've always been healthy, and my energy level was high.

The findings came as a shock. I saw my husband's look of disbelief as he struggled to keep his composure. Surgery would be the next day. At least I didn't have much time to worry about it, because I was busy with my list of pre-op directions. Having said this, I will admit the only direction that was hard for me to follow was getting a good night's sleep; it just didn't happen. This was all too new, too unbelievable!

• •

The flurry of activities at the hospital the next morning proceeded smoothly, and I felt surprisingly relaxed while waiting in my not-quite-designer hospital gown and long surgical stockings. I had two sedatives: one was given through the IV, and it helped some. The other came from my heart, and it helped a lot. This one was a line from the Twenty-third Psalm that kept running through my head. *He makes me lie down in green pastures.* I repeated these words over and over in my mind as the clock ticked down to operating room time, and they gave me courage and comfort. Even in surgery, with the oxygen mask over my nose, those words calmed me as I pictured myself resting in a quiet, safe, and serene place. Thank God for Sunday school and memorizing Bible verses! Thank God for holding us in His hands when we have to let go completely and trust ourselves to the care of others.

A few hours later, waking up in my hospital room, I had an IV port on each wrist, a catheter in my bladder, an uncomfortable NG tube through my nose into the stomach, and an eight-inch incision in the abdomen. When the nurse asked me how I felt, I remember telling her that I felt "very cozy." I know this was largely due to the presence of my husband beside me holding my hand, but also due to those comforting lines from the psalm that kept me from being afraid.

Whatever comes, I know that those green pastures will continue to refresh and renew my spirit and will provide a sweet respite whenever fear grabs my heart. *He makes me lie down in green pastures.* Yes!

Do scary thoughts sometimes tempt you to lose faith? When that happens, try meditating on this comforting scripture, breathe deeply, and picture yourself in a place of rest and peace. Your own Angel Hug will always be as close as a prayer.

When a train goes through a tunnel and it gets dark, you don't throw away the ticket and jump off. You sit still and trust the engineer.

CORRIE TEN BOOM

Father, there is such great comfort in these beautiful verses from the Twenty-third Psalm. How I love the peacefulness of Your green pastures! I expect someday to be in the midst of life's hustle and bustle again, but today I rest gratefully in this quiet place, filled with Your love and peace. Thank you! Amen.

Are You Going to Play It?

. . . .

My grace is sufficient for you, for my power is made perfect in weakness.

2 CORINTHIANS 12:9

My husband and I like to play pinochle. Bidding and trying to make one's bid are challenging and fun. My husband, who is probably the better player, is more conservative, while I often overbid, expecting to find just the cards I need in the three-card "blind" that is awarded the bidder. When we turn over the blind and it's pretty obvious I won't be able to make it, my husband often asks, "Are you going to play it?" An option in pinochle is to throw in the cards, subtract one's losses, and deal the next hand.

When cancer becomes a reality for us, we also have an option. We can throw in the cards and give up, or we can pick up our imperfect hand and play it for all it's worth. Somehow, I believe playing it is the more honorable (and certainly the more courageous) way. "Throwing it in" gives in to defeat and shuts out any chance for victory, however small that chance might be. Aside from that, I think we owe it to our loved ones to be strong, to be examples of faith, and to demonstrate courage, because tough times are going to come to all of us, whether in the form of cancer or some other difficult experience. Aren't these the attributes we've always

. . . .

admired? The world never has enough role models for positive attitude; now you have a golden opportunity to provide one. With God's grace, you can do this!

I once knew a woman who was terribly crippled by arthritis. As an elder in the church, I was assigned to visit her every week. I confess I dreaded that first visit because I didn't know her very well, and I was not sure how effective I would be in cheering her up. Was I in for a surprise! Marie had an impish smile on her face and a twinkle in her eyes. She was absolutely thrilled to have someone to talk with, and she did love to talk! She told me about her family, the football team she liked to watch on television, and how thoughtful the nurses were at the nursing home where she lived. Her hands were so crippled they were useless to her, but she didn't let that steal her happiness. As my visits continued each week, she never flagged in enthusiasm and once, in her exuberance for conversation, she told me if I needed to leave I'd better go or she would "talk my arm off." It could easily be said life hadn't treated her fairly, but she hardly seemed to notice. Instead, she became a blessing to everyone who walked into her door, so that the person who came to console really gained the consolation. It's nice to get Angel Hugs, but it's even nicer to pass them on to others.

OK, I've been dealt a bad hand. Am I going to play it? Yeah, I am. I'm going to give it my very best shot, even if there's only the slightest hope of winning, because when it's all over, whether three years from now or thirty, I know whose arms will catch me. You've been dealt a hand, too. How about you? Are you going to play it?

Our greatest weakness lies in giving up. The most certain way to succeed is always to try one more time.

THOMAS EDISON

Lord, I realize life is not a game, and it isn't a dress rehearsal. It's the real thing. Please help me use my time wisely. I feel Your love all around me today. Thank You for that love, and thank You for the gift of this day! Amen.

The Gift of Being Needed

• •

*Carry each other's burdens, and in this way you will
fulfill the law of Christ.*

GALATIANS 6:2, NIV

Before my cancer diagnosis I was heavily involved in
volunteer activities and kept a very busy schedule. I
remember one particularly stressful day, several months
ago. My schedule had included an 8 a.m. breakfast
meeting, a 10 a.m. appointment, a 2 p.m. committee
meeting, a 4 p.m. board meeting, and my book discussion
group in the evening. Further, my ninety-year-old mother
had just moved into a rehab center after breaking her
hip, and I popped in at the center whenever I could
squeeze in a few minutes. My stress built as the day
passed, and when I wheeled Mother's chair back to her
room after dinner, she remarked that I looked as if I had
a headache. She always had the ability (which I hated as
a teenager!) to know what was going on with me, but
when she offered to rub my shoulders and neck I
automatically started to say, "Oh, no, that's all right."
Then it flashed through my mind that she really wanted
to do this, so I just smiled and said, "Oh, yes, that would
be lovely!"

I moved my chair so that my back faced her
wheelchair, and as she lifted her thin, frail hands to rub
my neck I was thankful she couldn't see my face because
tears were flowing from my eyes. Her butterfly touch
didn't do much for my muscles, but the love in that touch

• •

evaporated my stress. My father had died a year earlier, and since that time, Mother's fragile health required round-the-clock care. Daily she is bathed, dressed, cooked for, lifted in and out of bed, and sometimes spoon-fed. Not by her own choice, she has had little opportunity to do things for anyone else.

As her feather-light touch melted away my stress, I was reminded of a basic aspect of human happiness. *We all need to be needed.*

As long as I live, I will never forget this precious gift of love my mother gave me. She will probably not walk again, she may not live long; yet even in this condition she gave me a huge Angel Hug and I, who needed her touch so much, inadvertently gave her the gift of being needed.

There may be friends or neighbors who call you and ask how they can help. I've had offers to help me run errands, to bring food, or to take me to radiation treatments when my husband couldn't be there. You probably have, too. Don't be too quick, or too proud, to deny someone this opportunity. One thing that is really helpful is to have a friend go with you to the doctor and take along a notebook or tape recorder to help you remember what the doctor says. Try as we might, it's hard to remember everything when we think about it afterwards. Getting groceries or items from the drugstore can be a huge help, too, so when a friend calls, tell her how much you would appreciate her help in picking up a few things. Write your list and keep it handy so you will be ready.

Give all you can, but remember there are times to step back and let someone else feel needed. Maybe that time is today.

The love we give away is the only love we keep.
ELBERT HUBBARD

What a blessing, Father, to share time with people I love! Please make me sensitive to their needs, whether they need to be comforted or to comfort me, whether they need my strength or whether, at times, they need to give strength to me. Keep me tuned in so I can recognize their needs and not think only of my own. Amen.

Eating over the Sink

> *Thou preparest a table before me in the presence of my enemies: thou anointest my head with oil, my cup overflows. Surely goodness and mercy shall follow me all the days of my life; and I shall dwell in the house of the LORD for ever.*
>
> PSALM 23:5–6

When my mother-in-law became a widow after nearly fifty years of marriage, she lost more than a husband. She lost much of the will to keep up her activities in the usual way. One way this manifested itself was that she would not cook regular meals for herself. Usually, when hunger got the best of her, she walked over to the refrigerator, opened the door, and began a conversation with herself that went something like, "Now I wonder what there is left over that I could have a few bites of?" Rummaging around, she might come up with a few tidbits she would carry over to the sink. Grabbing a fork or spoon, she stood at the sink, looked sadly out her kitchen window, and ate her dinner of whatever she had managed to find. She hardly ever sat down to eat, which meant she didn't take time to make it look appealing for herself—pretty napkins, maybe some flowers, now and then perhaps her best china—but merely ate to satisfy her physical hunger while standing over the sink. For a woman who had devoted decades to the care of others (her sons and husband, then grandchildren and great-grandchildren), Ruth probably didn't stop to consider that she herself deserved care. I'm guessing many widows do the same.

I believe God wants more for us. I believe God wants to "prepare a table before us" by being part of all that we do, including our simple meals and household activities. When you are feeling fatigued because of your treatments, you may be tempted to skip meals or not sit down and eat. Please take those few minutes to set out the most appealing food you can find, and then take time to enjoy your food as much as you are able. Your favorite music in the background might help, or try changing your location: one time at the breakfast table, another in the dining room, outside on a sunny day, or even on a tray in front of the TV if a special program is coming on. Radiologists tell us that eating well is important, and sometimes they don't even want us to count calories! Check with your physician to learn what kind of diet you should follow, but please use this time to be extra kind to yourself. A sprig of flowers on your table is cheering and encourages you to eat. If someone is helping you with meals and menus, you could suggest that a colorful setting, or pretty seasonal place mats, might help your appetite. I've found that caregivers and loved ones are usually eager to do anything they can to help.

I think "eating over the sink" has an even deeper meaning. I think it means settling for less than the full life God has planned for us. It means giving in to discouragement and limitation when prayer and faith could lift us to a more positive outlook. It could mean being so full of our own problems and illness that we neglect to share meaningful, joyous time with friends and loved ones. And here's a word of caution: *Don't live cancer twenty-four hours a day.* You, as well as your spouse or other family members, should each do something you enjoy every day, even if it's just making a cup of hot chocolate. Do things that relieve the stress that can build up in a situation where everybody focuses exclusively on the cancer. Try to keep your family life as normal as possible.

I know it's difficult to be cheerful when the prognosis is uncertain. But we can always cling to our faith and trust in God for the outcome. I love the words of the scripture we read today: "Thou anointest my head with oil, my cup overflows. Surely goodness and mercy shall follow me all the days of my life; and I shall dwell in the house of the LORD for ever." You might want to put a marker in your Bible at this chapter (Ps. 23) so you can find it easily whenever you need a lift, because with those reassuring words, we don't ever need to be people who "eat over the sink," do we? *Bon appétit!*

> *The human spirit can endure a sick body, but who*
> *can bear it if the spirit is crushed?*
>   PROVERBS 18:14, NLT

You tell us in Your word, Father, that You want us to live abundantly. Help me really understand what this means as I go through the simple tasks of every day. Increase my vision, help me see the possibilities of joy and wonder You have in store for all of Your children, and to be ever thankful for this abundance. Amen.

Kindred Spirits

• •

A friend loves at all times.

PROVERBS 17:17

I just had a wonderful phone conversation with my friend Debbie from Minnesota. Debbie and I met about a year ago through mutual friends. I liked her instantly, but the thing that really brought us together is that we were diagnosed with cancer in the same week, about six months after we met.

Now I look forward to our conversations as we talk about our treatment and how we are feeling, as well as lots of other things. She agreed to let me share her story with you.

Some time ago, Debbie lost her mother, her father, and her brother all within a span of three and one-half years. This really hit her hard, because each death was heart-related and very sudden. She felt she didn't get a chance to say goodbye to them, and also that they didn't have a chance to do things they might have wanted to do if they had known their time was so short.

So Debbie said to the Lord, "I don't think I want to die suddenly like that. It was too hard on me when my loved ones did, and I don't want my children to have to go through that."

Shortly before her diagnosis, Debbie took a sudden fall. She remembers feeling as if someone literally pushed her down. A few mornings later, she awakened with severe pain and called her doctor. He was busy and couldn't see

• •

her, but another doctor did. He ordered X rays, which quite unexpectedly revealed the cancer. Surgery showed her cancer to be at stage four, relatively far advanced.

Debbie feels confident that things happened this way in order to give her some time, as she had wanted. She has had seven months now, and finds that every day is a blessing. She told me that before she got cancer, she wondered whether she truly had an appreciation for every day, but now she definitely does. She is thankful she can get up, shower, and take care of herself. She is looking forward to her daughter's wedding in a few weeks, and hoping to be strong enough to participate in it.

It was very comforting to talk to my friend about dying. People usually avoid this subject as if by ignoring it they can prevent death from happening to them, but death is as natural as it is inevitable. With Debbie, we both know that some day it will come for us and we both feel very strongly that in the meantime, for every morning that we awaken, we will grab on to that gift with both hands and a thankful heart.

We each shed a few tears during our conversation, but I felt so blessed for having talked to her. We strengthen each other and the love just flows through the phone wires. God has blessed me with this new friend, and this has enriched my life. I pray that she will have many mornings to wake up and be joyful. However many there may be, I know her influence and her witness will last for a very long time. I pray that her story will also bless you and encourage you to be thankful for every day you are given.

There is a sacredness in tears. They are not the mark of weakness, but of power.
They speak more eloquently than 10,000 tongues.
They are the messengers of overwhelming grief, of deep contrition,
of unspeakable love.

WASHINGTON IRVING

Father, I believe friendship and love last forever. Help me remember this when someone I love passes from my sight into eternal life and I feel lonely without them. Help me realize I can still treasure their friendship, and hold their memory like a bright treasure in my heart. What a blessing You give me through friends. Thank You! Amen.

6

Created to Be Beautiful

• •

> *Be beautiful inside, in your hearts, with the lasting charm of a gentle and quiet spirit which is so precious to God.*
>
> 1 PETER 3:4, TLB

There is a big house on a corner lot in our neighborhood. For several years I have driven past this house every day, and if I had any impression at all, I would say it was unattractive. Then one morning, after a snowfall, I drove by and was astonished by how beautiful the house looked! Suddenly it was very appealing and I was enchanted just looking at it. I don't know what the difference was. Maybe there had been clutter in the yard, or the landscaping wasn't quite right, but the soft, pure blanket of snow erased all of that. I could see that the architecture of the house was very good. *It was designed to be beautiful.*

This made me think about my own life. Each of us was designed to be beautiful, perhaps not in a physical way but with a spiritual beauty that glows from within and reflects love back to our Creator. Sometimes the clutter of poor choices, resentment, or bitterness hides that natural beauty. God's forgiveness, love, and grace can erase these things like a pristine snowfall, and let the true beauty of our souls shine through.

Remember that you are created in God's image, so you know the Architect is great! So what if you are decked out in a hospital gown? So what if you've lost all your hair? You can be a blessing, a big, warm Angel Hug, to everyone you meet today if you will let them see the beautiful person God made you to be.

Sometimes it helps to think of specific ways to accomplish what we want to do. How can we be beautiful today? If we try to analyze what we appreciate most about our "beautiful" friends, it might be the warmth of their smiles or the twinkle in their eyes. Maybe it's also the fact that when we are together, they *really listen* to what we say. Add to these things a kind, gentle voice and there goes that beauty scale, just skyrocketing! These qualities make the most ordinary face vivacious and appealing. Being interested in other people is so important, too! As we turn from inward directed to outward directed, we become more vibrantly alive and more available to others, including God.

Today you can be a beautiful person by speaking kind words to those who share your day. Forget about yourself and ask how they are doing, then really listen to what they say. Give someone a big smile! You will feel better and…guess what…you will truly radiate the kind of beauty that is so precious to God!

A thing of beauty is a joy forever…
JOHN KEATS

Lord, You are the only one who can look past my outward appearance to see what I am really like, who I really am. My heart's desire is that You will find me pure and beautiful within. You made me in Your image, and I know this is the way You want me to be, but I need Your grace every day to help me. Amen.

What Difference Does It Make?

● ●

> *But the fruit of the Spirit is love, joy, peace, patience, kindness, goodness, faithfulness, gentleness and self-control.*
>
> GALATIANS 5:22–23a, NIV

It's just beginning to snow outside, and I am remembering a wonderful, sunny vacation. My husband and I had lots of fun on our trip, but travel can be stressful, and one particular afternoon we returned to our motel feeling especially tired and harried. When we pulled into the parking lot, I gathered up a handful of maps and brochures and then spilled them all on the floor. Flustered, I got out and, sure enough, all of the slick, shiny brochures slipped out of my hands again onto the ground. When my husband, who was no doubt tired from driving all day, responded with *"What's the matter with you?"* I picked everything up and stomped into the motel. I didn't come back with a sharp answer; I simply sulked.

Lying awake in the middle of the night (isn't it funny how we can't sleep when we're angry or sulking?) I thought about my behavior and felt guilty. I'm a follower of Christ. I'm committed to a life of faith. Because of this, I believe I should respond better to the little frustrations of life. If I don't, what difference does my Christianity make?

It's easy to have a positive attitude when everything is going just fine. When our faith requires something

● ●

better from us is during those other times. Sulking is not the answer.

What difference has it made in your daily life? Has being a Christian helped you give a soft answer in a heated discussion? Has it given you patience in a traffic jam? Has it sweetened your words to a loved one when you didn't see eye-to-eye?

What about now? What difference does it make now when you face the biggest battle of your life? Is cancer bigger than our faith? No. Is cancer a reason for us to feel sorry for ourselves and sulk? I don't think so. Does it give us a unique opportunity to stretch our faith and lean on God in every distress? I believe it does. I have to believe that my faith will sustain me in this as it has in everything else up to this moment. I have to believe that God will hold on to me for dear life, and I am determined to keep the faith. I know Whom I have believed, and that makes all the difference.

In every success story, you find someone has made a courageous decision.

PETER DRUCKER

Lord, it is so easy to be cross and spiteful when things don't go the way I want them to, yet I know You expect more of me. I am Your child, and that reality makes my life wonderfully different. Help me remember this difference in all my relations with others. Amen.

Courage

> *When you pass through the waters, I will be with*
> *you; and when you pass through the rivers, they will*
> *not sweep over you.*
>
> ISAIAH 43:2, NIV

The weather is still cold and blustery, and I am longing for springtime, so I want to share another vacation story with you. Together we can soak up some sun, at least in our imaginations!

It was the kind of setting you'd have to call paradise: a cloudless sky overhead, white sailboats dotting perfect blue waters. Our family had spent the morning snorkeling from a small boat. As we shared lunch prepared by the captain's wife, we happened to mention that we are from Oklahoma. They told us that another couple from Oklahoma sometimes charters their boat. "You know, that guy is amazing!" the captain said. "He's a quadriplegic in a wheelchair, but he loves to snorkel."

Then the woman said, "We put the snorkel and fins on him and just toss him into the water! As you can imagine, he had to be pretty persistent the first time, but his confidence persuaded us, and he enjoyed it tremendously."

This story made a huge impression on me because I'm afraid of water. I can snorkel, but only with a life belt around my waist and while trying not to hyperventilate when I jump into the water.

It made me think about Peter—that impulsive, passionate, hot-headed (but dearly loved) disciple—when he tried to walk across the water to Jesus. His courage failed the moment he realized what he was doing, and he started to sink. We're in a similar predicament, aren't we?

At times our illness tends to overwhelm us and we lose courage. Sometimes the waters seem rough and we wonder if we, too, might sink. But just then, Jesus reaches out His hand to comfort and encourage us.

I am thankful for that unknown man whose amazing story I heard. His courage inspires me and makes me feel that I can face whatever I have to face today. His example shows me that God wants us to live with enthusiasm, not timidly or fearfully. Whatever it is we attempt, when we take the first step God is always there to hold us up.

My friend Helga was diagnosed with cervical cancer twenty years ago. (It's exciting to hear about a twenty-year survivor, isn't it?) She remembers being upset that her doctor called to give her the bad news while she was at work! The time passed slowly until her scheduled appointment, and she finally began her treatments. Her cancer was stage three going into stage four, so radiation was scheduled to try to shrink the tumor. Her radiation treatments ran from December until May, with three weeks on and then time off before starting again. When she was checked again, the tumor was very small. Her doctor felt this was partly because of her positive attitude. I know she also believes in prayer and has a strong faith.

Even though the tumor appeared to be gone, the doctor recommended surgery, expecting a 98 percent chance of cure. Now, twenty years later, we know that the cure was achieved.

Helga admits that at first she wondered, "Why me?" Then she followed the advice of a friend who encouraged her to pray for peace of mind, and she gave the problem to God.

Helga loves nature, and on nice days she sat outside and listened to the birds while reading her Bible. She feels she grew much closer to God during her illness, and firmly believes that this helped make her well.

I am sharing Helga's story because I want you to know that bad news can sometimes be turned around. Don't give up if you are diagnosed with a stage three or stage four cancer. Give your worries to God, work with your physician to bring about your best chances for a cure, and, finally, take courage. Medical specialists often stand in awe of the power of prayer, faith, and a positive attitude.

Bravery is falling but not yielding.

LATIN PROVERB

Father, I have met so many people who thrill and inspire me with their courage! I marvel at the story of the quadriplegic, and I long to have faith and boldness like his. Why should I ever be afraid? You have promised to be with me, and I cling to that promise. Whether in facing illness or leaping unafraid into the water, I know I can do all things through Christ who strengthens me. Thank You for this. Amen.

By Faith, Not by Sight

*So we are always of good courage… for we walk by
faith, not by sight.*

2 CORINTHIANS 5:6a, 7

My leg was in a plaster cast from foot to thigh because of
a fall that resulted in torn knee ligaments and surgery.
As the weeks dragged on, I looked forward to the day
the cast would come off and I would see my leg again,
hopefully as good as new.

I managed using crutches and forgot about the cast
for hours at a time, but sometimes my leg would tingle
and I wanted to scratch it, which was impossible due to
the cast. If you have never experienced this, please believe
me that nothing makes one want to scratch more than
knowing it's impossible! Also, I couldn't see my knee
healing or the ligaments mending. I had to have
confidence in the doctor's skill and trust that good things
were happening inside that cast.

Sometimes we face a problem for which we can't even
imagine a solution, and everything seems to go wrong.
We yearn for healing of our bodies and pray that the
radiation, chemotherapy, or medications we are taking
will work and, all unseen, heal us. We become tired and
impatient when the healing doesn't come as quickly as
we had hoped. Still, I believe God uses our trials to make
us strong and that He is working for our good, even when
the problem is frustrating like an itch that we can't
scratch! God will work through our doctors, through our

faith, and through the strength and support of our loved ones. And as happened with my leg in the cast, God strengthens and mends us when we put our trust in Him, even though we can't always see or understand how it works. When we can't see the way, life becomes a matter of faith.

This is how our friend John felt after being diagnosed with rectal cancer. His aggressive treatment included almost-daily trips to the doctor as he underwent radiation and chemotherapy treatments. During treatment, John trusted the professionals who cared for him, but the one thing that really carried him through was his belief that God was in control of his life. Even so, the post-surgical chemo sessions began to make him very ill, and the doctor could not seem to stop the nausea.

When thinking about how cancer has changed his life, John enjoys remembering the friends he made on the Internet. Through this medium, he was able to connect with others who were going through similar trials. In one case, after hearing of a new friend's brain tumor, John told her that he would be praying for her. She quickly informed him that she was an atheist and she was not going to have the surgery. Yet, he learned later that she did agree to the surgery, and that his words had impressed her. What a blessing for him to know that his prayers gave her a feeling of hope!

We never know how our encouragement, or sharing our faith, will affect others. For some, it can be a matter of life and death, and the difference between hope and despair. You may be the only person who can give that special Angel Hug of hope to someone today.

*All I have seen teaches me to trust the Creator for all
I have not seen.*

RALPH WALDO EMERSON

*Thank You, Lord, for the unseen but very real strength You
give me every day. Thank You for the skill and wisdom of
physicians, but even more for the miracle of Your constant
love and care. Amen.*

Tell Me What I Want

*But seek first his kingdom and his righteousness,
and all these things will be given to you as well.*
MATTHEW 6:33, NIV

It's almost Christmas, and I had hoped my treatments would be finished, but they are not. However, I am determined not to let this diminish the joy of the season! I've been busy with a minimum amount of shopping, while trying to conserve enough energy to get me through all the holiday activities.

Looking over my list, I come to Aaron, my youngest grandchild. He's a big boy of seven now, but last year, when he was six, his mother told me a cute story that really made me stop and think. It seems that when she asked Aaron what he wanted for Christmas, he wasn't prepared to answer. This in itself is surprising! But what surprised me even more was what he said. He hesitated a moment before saying, "I don't know. I guess I'll have to watch TV to find out what I want."

We are only too aware of the enormous and expensive campaigns carried out by toy manufacturers to plant ideas in the minds of children, to make them want certain things. It surprised me, though, that Aaron articulated it so clearly. This got me wondering if even we grown-ups sometimes rely on outside influences to tell us what we want instead of making judgments based on our own needs and wishes.

At this wonderful and holy season, I find my wants are quite a bit different from other years. As you no doubt know, cancer is a powerful reality check! It cuts through to the important stuff like love and values. My wish list is mostly just to be with my family, to hold them and hug them, to sit down at meals and cherish family traditions, as well as the special foods everyone contributes, such as my sister's fabulous Pink Arctic Freeze, without which our holidays would be incomplete.

My wish list also includes my mother being well enough to get bundled up and come to our celebration from the nursing home where she lives. For these things, I don't need to watch TV commercials to know what I want. Of course, I'm only human and my list (which my husband always asks for, so his typical Christmas Eve shopping will actually come up with something I will use and enjoy) also contains material things I think I would like to have.

Even if we must spend Christmas, or other special times, in the hospital, our wish list could be pretty easily filled by the smiling faces of people we love. It also helps to keep a tape recorder nearby so we can push in a cassette, press a button, and hear some of our favorite music right there in bed. When cancer rearranges life in surprising and difficult ways, our faith can help us see things more clearly than ever. The nice thing is we don't even have to watch the commercials to know what we want!

It is not how much we have, but how much we enjoy, that makes happiness.

C. H. Spurgeon

Father, as a mature person I should always make wise decisions, but sometimes my wants seem very childish. Please help me want those things that are uplifting, that will help me grow spiritually. And, Lord, bless all the children who touch our lives. They inspire us with their innocence, their honesty, and their whole-hearted love. Thank You for every one of them. Amen.

"For All the Things I've Done"

• •

Be kind to each other, tenderhearted, forgiving one another; just as God through Christ has forgiven you.

EPHESIANS 4:32, NLT

I hope you won't mind another little story about Aaron. He was about five years old, and he had been a trial for Mommy all day, whining for this and that, quarreling with his sister, and just being irritating in the little ways that drive mothers to distraction. Finally, she'd had it! She sent him to the playroom to play quietly and stay out of the way. His feelings were hurt, but deep down he understood why Mommy was upset. He was quiet for a long time, and when he finally came out of the playroom he walked over to his mother and handed her a piece of paper. His little face was serious and hopeful as he waited for her reaction.

Aaron had filled a big sheet of paper with hearts that he had drawn and then colored in. As young as he was, the motor skills to do this were not easy and his efforts represented a great deal of concentration and effort. As he handed her the paper, he said, "Here's for all the things I've done!" It was a peace offering and a love offering, his young heart full of repentance and yearning for forgiveness.

Aaron's mother was touched. Her reaction was a smile and a great big hug for her little boy. He broke into a big smile, too, knowing he was forgiven. Wouldn't you?

• •

This story made me think about our relationship with God. Try as I might, it seems that every day I fail in so many ways to live up to what God expects of me as a Christian. When I stop and think about it, I feel a lot like Aaron. I want to draw whole pages of hearts to offer to God when I ask for forgiveness, but He only wants one heart, a whole heart, from each of us.

Being ill gives us more time for reflection. We can draw hearts for God every time we show appreciation for those who care for us, and we can try to lighten the burden of our loved ones when they feel stress about our situation. We can try to understand what this feels like for our caregivers, and give our family more encouragement and consideration.

The wonderful thing is this: whenever we turn to God asking for His forgiveness and help, He gathers us up in loving arms just as Aaron's mother did, and the pain in our hearts instantly turns into a smile.

Houses are built of brick and stone, but homes are made of love alone.

AUTHOR UNKNOWN

Father, even on days when I act like a five-year-old spiritually, I know You still love me. I could paint a canvas the size of the sky and never draw enough hearts to show my gratitude! Your forgiveness and love overwhelm me because I don't deserve them at all. When You forgive me I feel clean and new, like a child who just ran outside in a spring rain. Thank You for the cleansing rain of Your love. Amen.

Living *A Christmas Carol*

• •

> *Cry out for insight and understanding. Search for
> them as you would for lost money or hidden
> treasure.*
>
> PROVERBS 2:3–4, NLT

One of the most delightful traditions we had when my
children were growing up was going, as a family, to a
production of Dickens' *A Christmas Carol*. We lived forty
miles from the theater, so the event had to be carefully
planned to fit in with an already busy season of school
band concerts and church activities, and some years it
just didn't work out. Whenever it did, we shared a
wonderful evening.

Remembering that, I was thrilled this Christmas to
be invited by my son John and his family to attend *A
Christmas Carol*. Our holidays this year were pared down
from the usual busy-ness because of my flagging energy
from radiation treatments, but I was certainly up to this!
Also, I found it immensely pleasant that John wanted to
share one of the special treats from his own growing-up
days with his children…and included me!

Several weeks later, when I was having a phone
conversation with John, I must have sounded a bit down.
I was feeling overwhelmed and uneasy about how my
life was going since I had had one metastasis of the cancer.
John's reply to that was so amazing it startled me, but it
gave me a wonderfully new way of looking at things.

• •

John listened to my little "pity party" remarks and said, "You know, it's a little bit like Ebenezer Scrooge. Scrooge had a whole new life after he had those dreams, with all the visits from Christmases past and so on. He completely changed his life and did all the good things he ever wanted to do. It was very liberating for Scrooge."

What a fantastic idea! I could hardly contain myself as I started thinking about all the really meaningful things I could be doing. I certainly don't want to be one of those people who come to the end of life and sadly think of all the things "*I wish I had done!*" Just think! I can do lots of them every day. None of us knows how many days we have. We read in the newspapers about young athletes dying suddenly in football practice, or even whole families in car crashes, but we don't expect that to happen to us. I don't mean to trivialize any kind of unexpected tragedies, but I'm just saying that time is limited and some day it will run out for everybody—not just cancer patients, but everybody. Isn't it a crime to be bored? Isn't every day just too absolutely precious to spend being depressed? Isn't it just sinful to neglect loved ones or let the wounds of a broken relationship go unhealed for even one more minute?

Thank you, John! And now I, like Ebenezer Scrooge, do pledge to one and all that I will henceforth live every day as fully as I possibly can. I will be liberated from selfishness and from meaningless things that steal my time, and I will give myself to things that really matter.

Not just at Christmas, but every day of the year, I am going to try to live *A Christmas Carol*. Will you join me? Angel Hugs are in store every day that we consecrate by giving joy to others, by living as fully as our energy allows, and by appreciating every new morning the way a changed Ebenezer Scrooge greeted that happy Christmas morning.

There is nothing like a dream to create the future.
VICTOR HUGO

I've always thought of Scrooge as a bad guy, so different from me, but when I take a closer look I see greed and selfishness in myself far more than I want to admit. With Your help, Lord, I am determined to care more for others and less about myself. You have blessed me so richly, how can I do otherwise? Thank You, Father, for speaking truth to us through people we love. Help me remember this lesson not only at the holy season of Christmas, but all year long. Amen.

Foundation Repair

• •

See, I lay a stone in Zion, a tested stone, a precious
cornerstone for a sure foundation;
the one who trusts will never be dismayed.

ISAIAH 28:16, NIV

My sister and I are getting our parents' house ready to
sell. Mother has been in the nursing home for sixteen
months, and we see many potential problems with an
unoccupied house. We have begun to sort through their
things. For a couple who were married sixty-nine years
and made very few moves, you can imagine how tough
an assignment this is!

The problem is compounded by the fact my sister
recently was diagnosed with a brain tumor, a suspected
metastasis from an earlier lung cancer, and is taking daily
radiation treatments. Her energy is low, but with the help
of our husbands, we are making progress on this
daunting task.

Just as we made final agreements on "who gets what"
and how to divide up Mother's original paintings among
her seven grandchildren, we discovered there are cracks
in the brickwork of the house. A structural engineer was
called, and his report showed we need serious foundation
repairs. By serious, I mean repairs that will cost several
thousand dollars. Our real estate agent has put the house
"on hold," and we have contracted with a foundation
repair company to shore up the sagging areas. This is a
complex procedure, and a pretty amazing one when you

• •

stop to think about it. That it is possible to lift an entire wall of a house built on a concrete slab is hard for me to comprehend. They promise a lifetime warranty, and we are on the schedule for next week.

I was lying awake last night thinking about this after reading my evening devotions, and it occurred to me foundation repair is a pretty wonderful thing! I believe every time we confess our sins and feel God's forgiveness, we experience a personal "foundation repair."

It could be said that the physical foundations of our "houses" are damaged right now, after cancer put some "cracks in the brickwork" of our bodies. But the great thing is, our doctors are skillful and dedicated, and they can shore up many kinds of problems. Beyond that, the deeper parts of our souls are renewed daily, without appointments or insurance forms, through God's love that gives us unfailing hope. Don't you just love the idea of that precious cornerstone laid by God? May these words comfort you and bless you today.

> *O, may this bounteous God through all our life be near us,*
> *With ever joyful hearts and blessed peace to cheer us.*
>   CATHERINE WINKWORTH

Lord, years ago I had a dream about building my house on the sand, and I believed that dream came from You. Thank You for caring enough to speak to me in so many ways... through Your Word, through other people, through the beauty of the outdoors, and even, sometimes, in dreams. I feel blessed to hear Your voice in these ways. Help me build my life on the sure Foundation of Christ. Amen.

• •

*Peace I leave with you, My peace I give to you; not
as the world gives do I give to you. Let not your
heart be troubled, neither let it be afraid.*

JOHN 14:27, NKJV

Most of the time when I've heard this scripture, it was
meant for the comfort of *someone else*. Now, when I read
these words and take them into my heart, they become a
precious comfort when I feel afraid or sick. I seem to hear
Jesus speaking them right into my own ear.

Since my cancer diagnosis, I've searched the Bible for
scriptures that bring peace and encouragement, because
even though I usually keep a positive attitude, fear and
anxiety come too frequently. I'm guessing you would
agree. It has been amazing to discover how many times
Jesus zeroed in on these things: peace, comfort, and
encouragement. He spoke to many important leaders as
well as the common people, and He was sympathetic
with their concerns because He knew that illness and fear
come to everyone, and that fear and anxiety rob us of
our life force.

What I'm learning is that peace, like happiness, is a
by-product of something else. We can't just decide to have
peace and, bingo, we have it, although a positive attitude
does help us find the things we believe in. Usually, peace
settles upon us in a soft, sweet way when we aren't even
looking for it. If we have been angry with someone, peace
may come when we resolve that conflict. If we have a

• •

difficult decision to make, peace may come when we face the problem prayerfully and then make the best decision we can. If there is someone we need to forgive, peace may come when we ask God to help us forgive that person. If we have tried to face our fears and problems all alone without turning to God, peace will come when we ask Him to help us.

I am glad peace isn't only for the successful, the wealthy, the strong, or the popular. Peace is a free gift for every one of us. It is the pillow that makes our slumber sweet and our dreams happy. Even when the prognosis is not good, we still have peace because our faith is stronger than fear, and faith lets our vision stretch far beyond what we can humanly see. My prayer for you is that God will richly bless you with peace every day you live. May every breath you draw be an intake of the peaceful, quiet strength that transcends physical stamina.

God cannot give us happiness and peace apart from Himself, because it is not there.
There is no such thing.

C. S. LEWIS

Father, I look around the world and see very little peace. Wars, economic turmoil, and the constant struggle of leaders for popularity and power make life stressful. Help me follow You quietly and simply, that I may know in my heart that true peace that passes all understanding. Amen.

The Will to Be Well

Everything is possible for him who believes.

MARK 9:23b, NIV

This scripture comes from the story of a man who brought his son to Jesus for healing. The son had been ill from childhood with an evil spirit that often threw him into convulsions. Jesus' response to the father, "Everything is possible for him who believes," may sound like a trite answer to our prayer for healing. On the other hand, the faith He asks for would stretch most of us to a level we have never experienced. But the amazing thing is that the father didn't just hand the boy over to Jesus and then take home a well child. The father became a *participant* by his willingness to believe.

We know that attitudes are critical in regaining our health. Even our treatments work better when we visualize positive results.

I practice visualization every day when I go to the radiologist's office and lie on the table for my treatment. The table is hard, the room is cold, and the big machine looming overhead seemed frightening at first. Now it's an old friend and I practice a little routine during each of the four doses of radiation. After the technicians put the shield in place (before they leave me and go into their "safe" room), I lie very still and let modern technology do its work. First, a dose on the front, with the machine right over my body. I breathe deeply and count "one thousand one, one thousand two, one thousand three, one thousand four, one thousand five, one thousand six," and the dose is over. Back in the room again, the technicians change the shield that will guide the next rays to a precise spot on my left side, the big machine moves slowly across, and I count again. Try it, but don't just count. Get tough! Be aggressive! Picture the beams as busy little scavengers searching out diseased cells and killing them. Then picture those cells shriveling up, completely powerless now and ready to be flushed out of your body. Picture your healthy cells taking only a tiny dose from the rays, a dose from which they will quickly recover before your next treatment.

After my four doses of radiation (front, both sides, and back), I try to keep positive thoughts going all day, visualizing the ongoing battle inside my body with the good cells staying strong and the diseased cells wasting away. If you are having chemotherapy, you can practice the same kind of visualization by picturing the medicine vigorously attacking the diseased cells and destroying them, while the healthy cells remain intact and strong. Try to actually *feel* the medicine working as it goes into your bloodstream. Picture yourself getting well from deep inside, one cell at a time, as you journey toward recovery.

Your prayer and meditation time is another great time for visualization. Get comfortable, close your eyes and breathe very deeply. Think of God's warm, healing love wrapping around you as you bask in His wholeness and goodness. As you breathe in and out, think about breathing in wholeness and breathing out sickness. Breathe in peace and breathe out pain. Take plenty of time, and don't let anything distract you. Picture yourself stronger and better every time you do this, and end with a prayer of thanks. This routine can be a powerful, daily Angel Hug that renews and sustains you. Many people have practiced this kind of Christian meditation with astounding healing results.

I don't know if it is God's plan to heal me and keep me cancer-free, or if for some reason it is not. I do know He wants me to trust Him and that He is trustworthy.

There is a light in this world, a healing spirit more powerful than any darkness we may encounter. We sometimes lose sight of this force when there is suffering, and too much pain. Then suddenly, the spirit will emerge through the lives of ordinary people who hear a call and answer in extraordinary ways.

MOTHER TERESA

Father, in my mind there is a picture of myself strong and healthy. Help me keep that picture in my mind as I move toward wholeness with the help of medical specialists, friends, loved ones, and, most of all, Your powerful healing spirit. Thank You for being as close to me as my very breath. Amen.

A Balloon for Grandma

• •

*Grandchildren are the crown of the aged, and the
glory of sons is their fathers.*

PROVERBS 17:6

Heather was only three when her grandmother died. The baby of the family, Heather had always been close to Grandma. Heather was very sad to lose Grandma, and she missed her very much.

Soon the time for Grandma's birthday came around, and Heather helped her mother choose flowers and a big balloon to take to the cemetery. Lovingly, the family placed the gifts at the tombstone and spent a few moments thinking about the loved one they all missed so much. Just as they were about to leave, the balloon, which had been weighted down with a small stone, fluttered up and away, instantly out of reach.

Heather was heartbroken that the balloon she had personally chosen for Grandma was gone. Big tears ran down her face, and she was inconsolable until her mother knelt beside her to explain something. "Honey," she said gently, "don't you remember that Grandma lives in heaven now? Look! Your balloon is on its way up to her right now so she can have it for her birthday."

Heather stopped crying. A smile lighted her tear-stained face as she watched the big balloon sail up high and out of sight. Now that she knew her gift had found its way to Grandma, she was happy.

• •

A similar experience was in store for Heather the next year in kindergarten. On Valentine's Day, everyone got a balloon on a string, and the children laughed as they ran, trailing them high above. Suddenly, the string on Heather's balloon slipped out of her small hand and was gone. She gave a gasp of disappointment, and then she remembered! When her friends came to console her about the lost balloon, Heather smiled confidently. "Oh, it's just gone up to heaven," she said. "Grandma's in heaven, and she really likes balloons."

Heather's story touched me with the trust and innocence of the little girl's faith. You and I each hold a balloon in our grasp. You might call that balloon our life. No matter how tightly we cling to it, some day, sooner or later, the string will slip out of our fingers and it will rise up out of sight. I'd like to think of that as a beautiful release, all sunlit and floating, like Heather's colorful balloon going home to Grandma.

And like Heather's, those tears will turn to smiles when the truth is gently explained to our loved ones and we soar free.

A happy family is but an earlier heaven.
JOHN BOWRING

I have a beautiful dream, Lord. My dream is that some day, after I am gone, when loved ones are together and the conversation happens to turn to me, their faces will brighten and they will laugh as they share happy memories. May their eyes light with joy, not tears, as they recall times we have shared. Dear Father, please grant that I may live so as to create this legacy—not for me, but for them—to leave sunshine and gentleness in the hearts of those I love. I pray this in Christ's name. Amen.

Gear Up!

. . . .

> *God…is able to do far more than we would ever dare
> to ask or even dream of—infinitely beyond our
> highest prayers, desires, thoughts or hopes.*
>
> EPHESIANS 3:20, TLB

It's Sunday evening, and I just returned from our ranch in eastern Oklahoma. The weather was beautiful and the stars, viewed without the distraction of city lights, were incredibly bright. For me, the weekend was a time of renewal and rejuvenation. This afternoon, five of us climbed onto ATVs (all-terrain vehicles) for a ride on gravel roads and across bumpy fields. This made me think of my youngest son, Joe, who is an expert on ATVs and motorcycles, both in riding them and repairing them.

I hadn't ridden since my surgery, and it felt a little strange at first. I was not confident about shifting gears, and finally noticed my four-wheeler was riding rough. Suddenly, the words "Gear up!" popped into my head. Sure enough, when I went to a higher gear the ride was smoother and I began to relax and enjoy it.

This made me think about the whole experience of cancer: the many doctor visits, the radiation or chemotherapy visits, all the visits to the pharmacist for medicine, all the phone calls and notes from friends who are wanting to encourage me. You know what I mean. I think it would be easy for one to get "stuck" in this and

. . . .

make a whole life out of our recovery. Yes, it's comforting to soak up all the attention and sympathy. The problem would be if we never moved beyond that. For me, it's time to gear up!

Gearing up will mean getting outside more. I walked at least five miles this weekend and it felt great. I know it made me stronger. Gearing up, for me, will mean thinking about being well, believing in the power of my body and all of those prayers for my healing. It will mean picturing myself strong rather than weak. It will mean being a participant and not just an observer in the business of life. Being on the four-wheeler, with the wind in my hair and the sun on my face, I felt fully alive. If, someday, another metastasis occurs, God's grace will help me deal with it. Until then, I plan to "gear up" every day and get right into the sometimes messy, sometimes fabulous, but always fascinating business of life.

I hope you are at this point, too. If you aren't well enough to physically be outdoors, I hope you will gear up emotionally. Spend more time thinking about others, and more time smelling the roses (or other flowers) that come into your room. Ask your loved ones to bring you some upbeat human interest story from the newspaper when they find one, so you can have a happy thought to reflect on throughout the day.

My prayer for you is recovery, and yet, even as I say this, I know that some day, for you as well as for me, cancer or something else will change everything. I have a feeling that when that time comes, I will once again hear those exhilarating words in my mind: *Gear up! There's a beautiful road ahead!*

Nothing great was ever achieved without enthusiasm.

RALPH WALDO EMERSON

Lord, sometimes the easy way is so appealing it's difficult for me to gear up, step on the gas, and take off. I'm thankful for the beauty of the outdoors, for the healing qualities of sunshine, rain, and gentle wind—all evidences of Your creative and sustaining love. Let Your dynamic energy renew me and lift me, at least temporarily, out of the routine of doctor visits, medication, and recurring illness. My heart is bursting with thanks for this exciting adventure! Lord, I want to gear up for life at its fullest and, if I forget, please send Your gentle wind and healing sunshine to remind me. Amen.

One Million Hearts

• •

As a face is reflected in water, so the heart reflects the person.

PROVERBS 27:19, NLT

My friend Joyce was diagnosed with an advanced and aggressive brain tumor, requiring immediate surgery. Afterward, her family moved her into a lovely hospice facility where her room was always bright with flowers and scented with her favorite perfume. Joyce had a lifelong love of flowers, and she was an artist with them, whether arranging them, making dramatic designs for her home, or wearing them with great aplomb. All of us who knew her considered her the epitome of a lady because of her gracious spirit, unerring sense of style, and most of all her warm, radiant smile. To imagine her lying in bed with her head partially shaved, drifting in and out of consciousness, was almost too much for me to bear.

When her husband called and asked me to take a turn sitting with her at the hospice, I said yes because I loved her and this seemed the least I could do. Still, part of me was dreading the moment when I would first see her, and wondering if I could carry on enough small talk to fill the hours and keep her entertained.

One thing I was determined to do was not cry. Well, that resolution went out the window the moment I stepped into the room. Joyce looked up, saw me, and her eyes lighted up. "I waited for you!" she exclaimed. As I

• •

rushed over to the bed to hug her, I couldn't stop the tears that flowed from my eyes. But you know what? It was OK. Joyce shed some tears, too, but what are a few tears between friends? She was not in a hospital gown, but in a silky pink gown, with her makeup on. This was true Joyce! As I sat beside her, she had so much to say that her words just tumbled over each other. She had never talked a lot about her religion, but suddenly she was telling me things I knew came from a special insight as God revealed Himself to her in wonderful, new ways.

Her husband told me she had asked him for a drink of water the day before, and when she tasted it she said, "Oh, not that regular water! I want some of that special water like I had last time." He was perplexed, but finally poured some sparkling water into a glass for her. Surprisingly, she was satisfied.

This reminded me of Jesus' parable of the living water, when He told the woman that whoever drank of it would never thirst again. I realized that part of Joyce was in a place I could not visit, partly in this world and partly in the next. Who was I to wonder if she had tasted living water?

She talked to me about her new house. She had a beautiful house and garden in Arizona, but this was someplace *really* wonderful she was thinking about. Again, I couldn't argue. All I could do was listen in amazement and know I was hearing something very special.

At the memorial service, Joyce's daughter, Michelle, said a few words I will never forget. She told about a visit she had with Joyce near the end. Michelle stopped on her way to work, and asked her mother to give her a thought for the day. Joyce closed her eyes for a moment before answering, "I can't. My brain is just too tired."

"Well, then," said Michelle, "give me just one word. Give me a word for today."

Joyce smiled into her daughter's eyes and said, "A million hearts. A million hearts of love." In the richness of that moment, Michelle knew her mother was giving her a benediction of love with every ounce of her strength. Michelle went out to face the day with the great peace that comes from knowing one is deeply and dearly loved.

Some day, we will all be in this position, between one world and the next. I hope my last words to my loved ones will give them the same courage, comfort, and unforgettable memories of those words Joyce gave her daughter, "A million hearts of love." I think I'd better start practicing today.

The heart that has been truly loved never forgets.
THOMAS MOORE

What a precious gift, Lord, to spend time with friends whose love and trust are such a blessing! I pray You will help me be the kind of friend who also blesses them. For those special friends who are now gone out of my sight, I give thanks for our time together. Their memories enrich my life. Amen.

Diamonds in Ashes

The Spirit of the Lord God is upon me, because the Lord has anointed me to bring good tidings to the afflicted… to give them a garland instead of ashes, the oil of gladness instead of mourning.

ISAIAH 61:1a, 3b

My mother became a bride in 1931, during the Great Depression. The ring my father slipped onto her finger was symbolic of a love that was destined to last seventy years, though neither of the young people could have guessed that. The ring was, indeed, more symbolic than valuable, with its tiny diamond. A few months later, this young couple who had enjoyed carefree evenings with friends and neighbors in the city suddenly faced a harsh reality. Like thousands of other workers, my father was laid off from his job. Finding another job was not possible, so my parents decided to return to his parents' farm, to live with them and work for them.

The move wasn't easy, but it was a good solution to their problem. One of Mother's duties was to remove the cold ashes and rake up the live coals in the wood stove every morning, then start another fire to warm the house. One morning, in stirring the ashes, Mother's ring fell off. She didn't notice it until later, and then, in despair, realized that her ring had been thrown out into the yard with last night's ashes. Although they searched desperately, the ring was never found. It was several years before they could afford another one.

I think we often throw away diamonds with the ashes of our lives. I know I've done it, and that realization is painful as I look back. When I made bad decisions that hurt people who loved me, I was throwing away diamonds with ashes. When I chose a busy social schedule that robbed my children of time they needed with me, I threw away diamonds with ashes. This is sorrowful for me. I'm sure you have your own memories and your own sorrows. Even though we pray about them, and even though we ask forgiveness from the people we hurt, we still feel bad whenever we think about it.

Having cancer is life changing in more ways than one. Surprisingly, some of these changes can make us better persons if we learn to see things clearly and to distinguish the true "diamonds" from the "ashes" of life. What matters is not what we've lost, but what we have left, and this is different for every one of us. When you take some quiet time today to talk to God, thank Him for all the things you have left. Some ideas to help you get started: you still have plenty of love to give and receive, an imagination to picture beautiful things, a memory to recall life's precious moments, friends who care about you, and hope for good things in your future.

Just because the ring is gone doesn't mean your finger is bare. You are still a cherished child of God and *that* diamond will last forever.

What oxygen is for the lungs, such is hope to the meaning of life.

EMIL BRUNNER

Sometimes it takes skill and discernment to tell the difference between diamonds and lumps of coal. Father, please give me that discernment, that I may pay attention to the important things while there is time. I would rather live with joyful memories than with bitter regrets. Amen.

Looking on the Heart

For the LORD sees not as man sees; man looks on the outward appearance, but the LORD looks on the heart.

1 SAMUEL 16:7b

My friend eagerly anticipated the birth of her first grandchild. This time, however, the joy of birth was clouded by a heart-breaking reality: the baby girl was born with severe birth defects.

My friend, a committed Christian, told me she paced the floor all that night, crying and praying, asking God how this could happen when she had trusted Him so completely. Her agonizing prayers finally brought peace and a new clarity, as God put these words into her mind: "I want you to learn to see as I see, to look on the heart and not on the outward appearance."

This word from God comforted my friend. Today, several years later, the child is bright and thriving, surrounded by a loving, supportive family.

It's easy to read profound lessons in the Bible without internalizing them, but not nearly so easy when we are put to the test. You and I are being put to the test right now. Surely, the least I can do in my Christian walk is to look upon the heart of everyone I meet, to see each person as a child of God and not judge by outward appearances.

Cancer seems to have a leveling effect, so those of us who are recovering or in treatment together form a bond that is amazingly strong. We encourage each other; we wipe each other's tears; we rejoice over every new level of wellness. When we do get well, we will probably have lots of new friends and a broader outlook on life because of those who shared this road with us.

Healing goes far beyond the physical body. I wonder what God sees when He looks on my heart. If He sees anger or resentment, He is seeing a disease that can't be cured by medical specialists. These "life defects" can rob us of happiness and take away our self-confidence.

You're already going through the toughest assignment, facing cancer. When you finally walk out of the doctor's office with a great report and no more appointments, you won't want to be weighed down with old baggage.

Letting go of resentment can make our healing complete, and it's as simple as a prayer. Remember this, too: if someone has hurt you, forgiving that person goes a long way toward healing.

What does God see when He looks at me?

God made you as you are to use you as He planned.
S. C. McAuley

Loving Father, please help me to always be compassionate. I pray that I may never grieve You by carrying resentment in my heart. If I sometimes feel I've been treated unfairly, please forgive me, for I know I have been richly blessed. Help me live so that what You see in me is pleasing to You. Amen.

A Season for Everything

There is a time for everything, and a season for every activity under heaven.

ECCLESIASTES 3:1, NIV

It was early spring and I was planning a birthday dinner for my stepdaughter, Kathy. Oklahoma weather is notoriously fickle, and this year was no exception. Nevertheless, I was determined the house should look nice for Kathy and our guests, so I went to the garden store and bought some beautiful hibiscus plants to set out by the front door. They were lovely the day of the party when the sun was shining, but late that night the wind increased and temperatures fell below freezing. So there I was, out in the yard at 11 p.m. in my robe and slippers, trying to fit plastic bags over the plants. Opening thin plastic bags in the cold wind was very difficult, but the real problem was I was trying to force the season to be something it wasn't.

Sometimes we fail to appreciate the seasons of life, or try to force them to be different than they are. Who wants to be old, when society focuses on youth and beauty? Yet we know every birthday is a gift from God, and this seems especially true now that cancer has become an unwelcome part of our lives. Yet here's where we're planted, so I think the best thing we can do is make today the best it can be, just cramming it full of thankfulness and a strong faith that God will use us and help us make this season meaningful.

I told you about the hibiscus plants, so now I'll tell you, as Paul Harvey would say, "the rest of the story." While the beautiful plants made a nice welcome for our party guests, they didn't survive. I'm not very good with plants, always assuming they will stay as beautiful in my garden as they are in the garden store or in those fabulous seed catalogues, but that seldom happens. I learned it isn't enough just to purchase the plant and set it out. Plants require care and knowledge on our part, as well as the proper amounts of sunshine, water, and warmth. The next time I planted hibiscus, I waited until the season was right. Delaying our pleasures is sometimes good for us and in this case, it was *very* good for the flowers! Yes, it's hard to accept the seasons when we long for spring and it's still winter, or when we become nostalgic for youth and miss the delights of maturity. Thank God today for this season of your life, whatever your age may be. Remember, you are exactly the age God made you, so it must be great!

When you were born, you cried and the world
rejoiced.
Live your life in such a way that when you die,
the world will cry and you will rejoice.

AUTHOR UNKNOWN

Here I am, Lord, not so young and not so old! I'm right where You put me in the great march of time. Thank You for giving me this moment of this day, this month, and this year. With Your help, I'll make these moments count for something good. Amen.

• •

In peace I will both lie down and sleep; for thou
alone, O LORD, makest me dwell in safety.

PSALM 4:8

Are you having trouble sleeping? Many nights, I find I
do. Even when I feel peaceful and calm at bedtime, the
midnight hours sometimes bring frightening thoughts
and restlessness. My husband tries to be patient, but
occasionally my tossing and turning get the best of him
and he asks me to please try to lie still. Of course, trying
to lie still makes it really hard to do! I've tried tricks, like
counting backwards from one thousand, or going
through the alphabet trying to think of a name beginning
with every letter, usually to no avail.

I've discovered sometimes I can get a fresh start by
turning the pillow over to the cool side, that smooth side
that isn't all wrinkled up by my fitfulness. Like climbing
into a fresh, smooth bed, the cool side of the pillow gives
me a second chance to relax and fall asleep.

A fresh start is always exciting. It's like taking a clean
sheet of paper to begin writing a report. Totally free from
errors and marks, the paper is perfect…like a plump,
smooth pillow.

When we are ill, contact with others is one of the best
ways to get a fresh start. When I am preoccupied with
my problems, I can't see past the end of my nose to
recognize the problems of someone else, and wallowing

• •

in self-pity really wrinkles up that old pillow! The best way to get that "cool side of the pillow" feeling is to consciously release my problems and think about something—or someone—else for a while. Mentally stepping away from our illness can be refreshing and sometimes worth more than a good nap! I don't mean that we should be unrealistic and pretend things are perfect, but we definitely can be more outward directed in our thinking. Any support group will point this out, because when we share our stories, our fears, and our successes, we really begin to care about others.

Physically, finding the cool side of the pillow might mean trying a different sleeping location, or getting a new, wonderfully soft pillow or blanket. Emotionally, it means releasing our fears to the Lord and finding the quiet peacefulness only He can give, peacefulness that smoothes out the wrinkles created by our anxiety. This is my hope for you.

I have read in Plato and Cicero sayings that are very wise and very beautiful;
but I have never read in either of them, "Come unto me all ye that labor and are heavy laden and I will give you rest."

SAINT AUGUSTINE

Father, I haven't thanked You enough for the many comforts of my life. Even in this time of illness, Your blessings are so abundant! For the house in which I live, for doors that keep me safe from harm and yet are open to friends, for sturdy floors under my feet, for clean, fresh water at the turn of a tap, for my comfortable bed, soft pillows, and cozy blankets. What luxury! I pray for the millions of people in the world who do not have these blessings, that somehow they may find rest tonight. May Your loving kindness wrap all of us in peace. Amen.

Laughing Out Loud

- -

> *A word aptly spoken is like apples of gold in settings of silver.*
>
> PROVERBS 25:11, NIV

Do you have a friend who always makes you laugh? I do, although this is a person with whom I have also shared life's inevitable sorrows and tears, because we have been friends for many years. But we do love to laugh, and sometimes we giggle like teenagers. One of the greatest character descriptions I ever heard, and one that I just love, was when my daughter Lori, who has known my friend all of her life, said, "Whenever I think of Ellen Jayne, I picture her laughing."

What a great way to be remembered! I'm sure you have friends like this, and I suggest that you spend as much time as possible with that friend (or friends) now while you are fighting cancer. Even when you don't feel well and might want to withdraw from the company of others, it is very important to stay involved with people.

I have learned from conversations with many cancer patients and survivors that laughter is one of the most powerful medicines. (If you've just had abdominal surgery you will have to settle for grins for a while and save the hearty laughing until you heal.) Laughter fills many of our deepest needs better than medical prescriptions, especially when shared with someone we love.

- -

Besides helping our blood pressure, easing depression, helping us forget pain, and reducing tension, laughter helps our food digest better. And surely you know that a smile instantly makes you better-looking! Sounds good, doesn't it? In fact, it sounds good enough to deliberately *look* for reasons to laugh. You might ask a friend to bring you a joke every day. If there are children in your family, they will love an opportunity to try their "knock-knock" and other jokes on you. They may forget the punch line, but they laugh so heartily at their own jokes that it is always delightful.

Think about silly songs that make you smile. Every generation has songs with rather zany lyrics. For good reasons, these songs seem to be most popular in difficult times such as war and economic depression.

You may be thinking cancer is serious business and not something to be laughed at. You're right, it is serious. Mother Teresa's work in Calcutta was serious, too, and yet when someone asked her what qualities were needed if one wanted to work alongside her, she replied, "the desire to work hard and a joyful attitude." In difficult and painful work like hers, we see the truth in the old Chinese proverb that one joy scatters a hundred griefs.

I believe God honors our prayers when we ask Him to help us find ways to smile or laugh. Laughter and tears are natural parts of life and both are sacred.

Now, if you really want to be joyful today, try to make other people laugh, too. Try it and see how many smiles you can coax out of a grumpy person, even on a Monday morning.

So be glad when that special, quirky friend comes to visit—and get ready for a joyful, health-giving laugh.

The most wasted day of all is that on which we have not laughed.

SEBASTIEN CHAMFORT

Father, people might think I'm strange to be laughing when there is so much need, so much want, and so much sickness all around. Yet, You have put within my heart a hunger for happiness and a longing for laughter that seem to resonate in the air like a prayer. I know there will be time for tears, Lord, but today I feel Your smile upon me like warm, dancing sunlight and I am smiling, too. Thank You! Amen.

Women of Grace and Courage

*Be strong and courageous! Do not be afraid of them!
The LORD your God will go ahead of you. He will
neither fail you nor forsake you.*

DEUTERONOMY 31:6, NLT

Since my cancer diagnosis, I have met so many people who are going through tough times, and so many who have gotten well against all odds, I am truly inspired. I want to share a few of their stories because I believe they will help you, too.

Even with regular mammograms, Barbara's breast cancer went undetected for several years. When she discovered a lump, tests showed a malignancy and she began the long road to recovery that included surgery, many months of chemotherapy, reconstruction, and weeks of radiation.

Barbara could have become angry and bitter, but she decided to *make a difference*. After her recovery, she dedicated herself to finding ways to educate and support others affected by breast cancer. Her vision and commitment have made a difference for thousands of women through Grow for Life, a cancer research and education foundation she helped organize.

Another woman of courage is my friend Judy. She surprised me by saying having breast cancer was the best thing that ever happened to her! (Wait a minute! Did she just say what I think she said?) Then she explained that her greatest fear had always been getting breast cancer, because she felt if that happened she would be a "big baby," but when it actually happened she was very calm and very brave. Having cancer made Judy appreciate the beauty of life, as well as understand the sudden changes that can come, altering everything in a single moment. She feels grateful for friends who stood by her and really cared. This made Judy realize how every gesture of compassion and friendship helps someone, and she believes this has made her a kinder person. Judy's story is a great example of God's grace upholding us and making us strong when we thought we were weak.

Another survivor, Ruth, recalls that when the doctor came to her room after her biopsy and said, "You have cancer," she was shocked.

"We think it will never happen to us," she said. She told the doctor she wanted a lumpectomy, and she wanted to know what her options were.

"You don't have any options," he told her. "You will have a mastectomy and it has to be tomorrow."

Waking in the hospital the night after surgery, Ruth saw a band of gold light coming down through the ceiling of her room. Bubbling up in the gold light were lots of tiny angels. She raised herself up to see if she was dreaming, but she was awake and the light was still there. When she told her family about this the next morning, her daughter said, "The angels came to tell you it isn't your time yet!"

Angel Hugs come in many different ways to bless and comfort us. Usually these ways are very ordinary, but other times they can only be called miracles.

Don't be afraid to take a big step if one is indicated.
You can't cross a chasm in two small jumps.
DAVID LLOYD GEORGE

Thank You, Father, for giving us strength even when we think we are weak. Thank You for Your grace that is far above anything we could ever hope or imagine. Thank You, also, for friends who challenge and inspire us. Help me put my trust in You today and every day to come, so that whether I am weak or strong, Your grace will uphold me. Amen.

25   The Gift of Encouragement

● ●

> *Therefore encourage one another and build each*
> *other up, just as in fact you are doing.*
>
> 1 THESSALONIANS 5:11, NIV

I was a piano teacher while my four children were growing up, which was nice because I could use my music education and still be at home with my family. Altogether, I taught more than two hundred students, and sometimes I wonder how many of them still play. I hope the experience of piano lessons enriched their lives and encouraged them to appreciate music.

You have your own sphere of influence, and it probably reaches farther than you imagine. Remember, even though your activities may be "on hold" right now, you can still be an encourager!

Most of us are getting extra amounts of care and concern now, but we still may occasionally fall into a slump. A few nights ago when I was saying my prayers, I asked God to forgive me for my discouragement, and then was immediately surprised by my words! I don't know where that idea came from, because I've never thought of discouragement as a sin, although when we are discouraged we're not trusting God unconditionally.

Do you know someone whose presence always makes you feel good? Someone who really listens to your ideas and then makes you believe you could go right out and conquer the world? That person has the gift of encouragement!

● ●

I want to tell you Gennie's story, and how her family encouraged her. After her mastectomy and chemo treatments, Gennie discovered one day that her hair was coming out by the handfuls. Her son called on the phone just then and he could tell that his mother was crying, so he asked what was wrong. She told him her hair was coming out, and she would have to start wearing a bandana. She invited him to come for dinner the next night and, to her surprise, he showed up with a bandana on his head! The second surprise was that her husband also came to the table wearing a bandana! She said her family had a lot of fun with this, and their sense of humor gave her encouragement and hope as they went through this difficult time together. I am very happy to tell you Gennie's treatment was thirteen years ago. Now, every Fourth of July, on the anniversary of her cancer diagnosis, her family celebrates with a cake and candles for the number of years since her surgery. Encouragement is powerful medicine!

Encouragement costs nothing except a kind heart, a listening ear, and positive words. No one is too old, too uneducated, too ill, or too poor to be an encourager. Even your smile can give encouragement to your caregivers, family and friends. Try to make sure your time together leaves them with hearts full of hope. Don't dwell on the downside, but on the exciting possibilities, no matter how remote they might seem. Hope and dreams are great flotation devices when we find ourselves in turbulent waters.

With all the attention from our friends and family, all of our medical appointments and treatments, and the research we do to learn more about our condition, we could easily be tempted to "make a career" of having cancer, but let's try not to do that. Today, let's put our health in God's hands and focus on encouraging others.

One of the most difficult things to give away is kindness... it is usually returned.

COURT R. FLINT

Father, I hear negative words all around me, but I don't want to speak that way or even think that way. Let me speak words that will help others move forward joyfully as they grow in faith. Thank You for giving me the opportunity to be an encourager to someone today. Amen.

Fill in the Hearts

• •

*The good man does not escape all troubles—he has
them too. But the Lord helps him in each and every
one.*

PSALM 34:19, TLB

The day after my cancer surgery, one of the nurses came
into my room and outlined two hearts on my bulletin
board. She explained to my husband and me that I was
to take two walks, very short ones at that point, and fill
in a heart for each walk I completed. My husband and
the nurse helped me up, and I sat on the edge of the bed
for a few moments gathering courage for those first steps.
Herman held my hand as we took those short, hesitant
walks, and he filled in the hearts when we got back to
the room. The next day, there were four hearts to fill in
and longer walks to take. I felt a real sense of
accomplishment when I completed each one.

I have thought about this several times. It is so
important to have someone's hand to hold when we need
help, someone to encourage and cheer us on when we
lack strength. At times, everyone needs a hand to hold.
Right now, we are probably on the receiving end of this
help, but with God's grace we will gain strength so that
some day we can offer a helping hand to someone else.
This is what brotherly love is all about.

I recently learned of a great example of brotherly love
that I'd like to share with you. A young priest from my

• •

home state of Oklahoma served for many years in one of the poorest parishes in Guatemala. Father Stanley Rother lived among the people, learned their language, built a clinic, taught the people to read, and provided spiritual guidance. He was adored by the people because they knew he really loved them.

When political conditions deteriorated there in 1981, it became unsafe for North Americans to remain in Guatemala, and U.S. citizens were called home. Conditions had become particularly dangerous for the Church, with six priests killed between May 1980 and July 1981. Typical tactics were to kidnap church leaders, torture them, and then kill them. Rother knew he was in danger. He returned to Oklahoma, but after a short visit with his parents he went back to the mission, knowing it might cost him his life. Tragically, he was murdered soon after his return, but his life and work left a lasting impression upon the people he had served, those poorest of the poor for whom Father Rother "filled in hearts" every day of his life with them.

You and I may never be called upon to lay our lives on the line in such desperate situations, but if we are I pray we will be strong and faithful. No matter who we are or where we live, there are always hearts to fill in and hands that reach out to us in need.

May God richly bless the persons who help us now when we need support, and may He also help us reach out to others as we become stronger.

The greatest use of life is to spend it for something that outlasts it.

WILLIAM JAMES

Father, I have heard the words "saints" and "martyrs," but they always seemed far removed. I am inspired to hear about someone who willingly gave up his life for others, for Your sake. I know there is work for me to do, too, and I pray for grace and strength to do whatever You ask of me, to help hearts that are hurting. Amen.

• •

> *There is a time for everything, and a season for every*
> *activity under heaven: a time to be born and a time*
> *to die, a time to plant and a time to uproot, a time to*
> *kill and a time to heal, a time to tear down and a*
> *time to build, a time to weep and a time to laugh, a*
> *time to mourn and a time to dance, a time to scatter*
> *stones and a time to gather them, a time to embrace*
> *and a time to refrain from embracing…*
>
> ECCLESIASTES 3:1–5, NIV

I hate to admit it, but I am a procrastinator. Actually, I have gotten better during the last few years and don't put off things quite as badly as I used to, but this is still a problem for me. Just think, if we had all the things accomplished that we intended to do before we became ill, if we had all those photo albums up to date and all of our closets perfectly organized, our slumber would be so much more peaceful! At least, mine would. I sometimes lie in bed at night thinking about the things I *should* have done, and while I make mental notes to get them finished, my stress level continues to build as I feel the urgency of the undone.

Yet we know many of those things aren't all that important. Who really cares if our closets and desk drawers are perfectly organized? We place an unnecessary burden on ourselves when we obsess over things that don't have lasting value.

• •

If there are things that have been worrying you, things you just haven't gotten around to doing, ask yourself this question: Is this something that will directly affect someone's safety, happiness, or well being? If so, you might want to ask a family member or trusted friend to help you get the project completed. If not, then it is probably something that would only impress people with your efficiency and orderliness, but not something worth worrying about. When you don't feel well and your energy is limited, it is nice to use that limited energy for things that really matter to you. For those "Type A" or obsessive persons, it may take lots of prayer to help you release your worries about undone things, turn them over to God, and let go. Wouldn't that feel good!

Procrastination is the art of keeping up with yesterday.

DON MARQUIS

I need help with my priorities, Father. My life seems cluttered with little problems that aren't worth my time or worry. Then I realize I have neglected other things that are really important. Give me wisdom to make good judgments and to do things when they need to be done. Amen.

I Think I Can, I Think I Can!

• •

Be strong and take heart, all you who hope in the
LORD.

PSALM 31:24, NIV

My friend Bob confessed that after the doctor told him he had prostate cancer, he didn't tell anyone for a whole year, not even his wife! He said he felt embarrassed, like someone who has fallen down and wants to get up quickly before anyone sees him. He admits he got worse by not telling about his illness, and this created his own depression. After telling his wife, Bob said he started to feel better.

Bob's doctor told him he had six months to one year to live. Now he wonders why people don't take a more positive approach. "It's like a meteorologist saying there's a 90 percent chance of rain, when he could say there's a 10 percent chance of sunshine," Bob said.

I understand, because when my doctor told me, matter-of-factly and without a trace of compassion, there was a 50–70 percent chance my cancer would come back, I was devastated. I know I would have felt better if she had said, "You know, you have a 50 percent chance the cancer won't come back!" Positive statements seem to bring positive results.

A year after his diagnosis, Bob (who, by the way, was still very much alive) felt he was finally "coming around" and stopped thinking he was about to die. He visited a support group, and his experience there points out

• •

another valuable lesson. At the meeting, he noticed everyone moping around and teary-eyed. Self-pity definitely prevailed.

Bob asked one, "Are you not feeling well?"

"Well, I have cancer." This was spoken indignantly, as if Bob should have known better than to ask.

"Everyone here has cancer," Bob said. Then he told the group, "This is my first meeting. I'm a florist, so I've been to lots of funerals. This is just like a funeral, and I'm not coming back, because none of you are talking about living; you're talking about dying."

It's very important to focus on the positive. Bob's attitude and keen sense of humor are so strong that when people tell him about their own cancer, they are surprised to learn that Bob has it, too. His theme is, "Celebrate life! It's a bonus!"

Bob said if we look at a picture taken one hundred years ago, those people are probably all gone now. If we could somehow see a picture taken one hundred years from now, all of us will be gone, too. "The important thing," he said, "is to enjoy life while we're here, to have a purpose, and to do something for someone else."

It took a year for Bob to learn how to handle his bad news but he made up for it by living exuberantly, and he has been an inspiration to many. He didn't blame God or become bitter; he simply celebrated every new day.

"I've had more dreams come true than I ever imagined!" he said.

Bob learned how to deal with bad news, and we know bad news comes to all of us at some time. I think every one of us should try to be like that fabled engine in the story we read as children, the engine that gave every ounce of its strength to accomplish what everyone else thought was impossible by confidently saying over and over, "I think I can, I think I can!"

> *Courage is the first of human qualities because it is*
> *the quality which guarantees all others.*
> WINSTON CHURCHILL

Sometimes, Father, the mountain in front of me looms so high I feel intimidated, and I'm tempted to give up. Then I remember You have promised to be with me. Yes, Lord, I believe the two of us together can do this! Thank You for leading me, loving me, and giving me courage to reach the top. Amen.

What 's Written in Your Heart?

• •

*I have hidden your word in my heart, that I might
not sin against you.*

PSALM 119:11, NIV

Several years ago, my two-piano partner and I prepared
an hour-long concert of Christmas music, all memorized.
One of the places we performed this was at my church.
Afterward, a friend came up to us and said, "If either
one of you were in an accident and got hit in the head, I
don't think any blood would come out, but only music
notes!" Her idea made us laugh, but truthfully I've often
wondered what it would be like if we could really see
inside our own minds. The Scottish poet Robert Burns
must have had that thought when we wrote about "seeing
ourselves as others see us."

We know that God sees into our hearts and minds. If
not, our prayers would just be meaningless words with
nowhere to go. It's easy to present a false impression to
acquaintances, and sometimes even to ourselves if we
aren't being honest, but the only thing that really matters
is who we are and what we believe deep down inside.

Since I first had cancer, I've done lots of soul-
searching. I imagine you have, too. I've tried to look at
my life objectively and ask myself if I'm really where the
Lord wants me to be, if my life is pleasing to Him. I also
wonder if I am being a good example to my loved ones,
because they, too, will need help and inspiration when
they encounter difficult times.

• •

When I was in elementary school, some friends and I wrote notes to each other with "invisible" ink. What we did was squeeze some lemon juice, dip the ink pen into the juice, and create our very secret messages. They could be read only by holding the paper close to a candle, where the heat darkened the dried juice and made the words visible.

I hope we aren't writing on our hearts with invisible ink. I hope whatever good words we have to share with the world will be real and true, preferably in bold font!

In the beautiful children's story, *The Velveteen Rabbit*, by Margery Williams, the Velveteen Rabbit asks the old Skin Horse about becoming real, and asks whether it hurts.

"Sometimes," said the Skin Horse, for he was always truthful. "When you are Real, you don't mind being hurt.

"Generally, by the time you are Real, most of your hair has been loved off, and your eyes drop out and you get loose in the joints and very shabby. But these things don't matter at all, because once you are Real, you can't be ugly, except to people who don't understand."

If we are truly going to be God's children, we have to be real even if it *does* hurt—and sometimes it will. God sees the real part of us, anyway. When we live faithfully and close to Him, the face we show the world will reflect our true heart, pure and whole, the way God created us to be.

A man that seeks truth and loves it must be reckoned precious to any human society.

FREDERICK THE GREAT

Some of the words I have written on my heart, Lord, are false and impure, yet I want to be true and clean. As I pray for healing and strength in my body, I also pray for a renewing of my heart, that I may be real in all of my relationships, especially in my relationship with You. Amen.

Are You Leaning Today?

• •

*The eternal God is your refuge, and underneath are
the everlasting arms.*

DEUTERONOMY 33:27a, NIV

Anthony Showalter, a Presbyterian layman, wrote the
words to the great old hymn, "Leaning on the Everlasting
Arms" in response to hearing from two close friends who
had lost loved ones. Showalter sent letters to his friends,
sharing the encouraging words of Deuteronomy 33:27,
and was later led to write a hymn based on that verse.

Are you leaning today? Is this one of those days when
you don't feel you can make it alone? The Everlasting
Arms are still available. Everlasting is a great word, isn't
it? Scholars believe the book of Deuteronomy was written
around 1406 B.C. and that the author for most of it was
Moses. So those words have been around for a very long
time. Just think of the countless people whose faith and
confidence have been restored by hearing these
comforting words!

"Leaning" days are good days to spend quietly in
the care of those special people around you. Perhaps it
would also be a good day to read some favorite Bible
verses together, or to simply enjoy clasped hands.

Families are all about sharing, too, and in every family
there are times when one or another needs special care.
When we help each other, providing loving support as it
is needed, we develop a close bond that no one outside
the family can ever fully understand or appreciate.

• •

I remember the day my daughter Lori was teaching her younger brother John to ride his bicycle. Lori is four years older than John, so by the time he was ready to graduate from training wheels to a real bicycle she was eager to be his coach. I can still see the two of them in my mind's eye. There they were on the neighbor's driveway (which had just the right amount of slope), with Lori holding on to the back of the bicycle. She gave it a push, then let go as John pedaled furiously, weaving a little from side to side but trusting that his big sister was near at hand and wouldn't let him fall. After several tries, John got the feel of it, and Lori stood back and watched. His face was beaming and hers was, too. I believe the bond between the two of them was strengthened at that moment. Helping someone gives us a nice feeling. Remember that when someone offers to help you. It can be an Angel Hug for both of you.

Life is short, and we never have too much time for gladdening the hearts of those who are traveling the dark journey with us. Oh, be swift to love, make haste to be kind!

HENRI FRÉDÉRIC AMIEL

Father, sometimes I feel embarrassed when I need the help of others. In my heart I know I shouldn't feel this way, but I need Your love to reassure me. I am thankful for the Everlasting Arms that are always available, every minute of every day. Even though I am leaning today, I feel faith and hope rising inside me and I pray that some day soon I will be stronger. In Jesus' name. Amen.

I Have Decided

*Trust in the Lord with all your heart, and do not rely
on your own insight. In all your ways acknowledge
him, and he will make straight your paths.*

PROVERBS 3:5–6

When my son Mark turned four, my mother gave him
music for the little song, "I Have Decided to Follow Jesus"
for his birthday. Then, playing the piano, she taught him
the song and he sang it at my parents' church a few weeks
later. This was their first grandchild, and you know how
grandparents like to show off those little ones!

I think that song had a powerful influence on Mark's
life, and that his decision still holds true. To me, as a
parent, this is a wonderful Angel Hug!

Having cancer requires you to make many decisions.
First, you must decide which doctor you will see for your
care. If surgery is required you must make a decision
about the hospital, and perhaps still another decision
about getting a second opinion. Insurance programs
require serious decision making, too. Choosing a
pharmacy is another important decision…some are
discount and can save a considerable amount of money,
while others are more conveniently located or offer more
friendly service. Sometimes, you will be asked to decide
which plan of treatment to follow. Even though your
doctor has recommendations, occasionally he or she will

ask you and your family to make the final decision when the course is unclear or the outcome uncertain.

During — and after — your treatments, you decide every morning when you wake up whether you will have a positive attitude or a negative one. You also make a very important decision, sometimes unconsciously, about getting well or not getting well.

Yet the most important decision we ever make is about our relationship with God, who created us and loves us. If we give Him top priority, other things will fall into place. We can lead full, meaningful lives serving the Lord whether we are ill or in perfect health. That part is not in our control, but what we can control is this: if we give ourselves away in caring for others and love God with our whole hearts, our lives will be meaningful and joyful.

Mother Teresa of Calcutta is a powerful example of one who gave her life for others because of the decision she made, her decision to serve the Lord. She said, "I try to give to the poor people for love what the rich could get for money. No, I wouldn't touch a leper for a thousand pounds, yet I willingly cure him for the love of God."

We make many decisions every day, and some are more important than others. Some are simple, like deciding what to have for lunch. Some are difficult, like guiding our young adult children into meaningful education and career choices. Even more important is deciding how to use the precious sixty minutes of each of the twenty-four hours we receive daily as a free gift.

My prayer for you is health and wholeness. May God hold you tenderly in the palm of His hand, and may His loving care watch over you always. In the words of the psalmist, may goodness and mercy follow you all the days of your life, and may you dwell in the house of the Lord forever.

> *Don't just live the length of your life,*
> *live the width of it as well.*
>
> DIANE ACKERMAN

Lord, I want to be one of the people who helps make things better in this world, who comforts the hurting and cheers the downcast, who shares what she has with the poor. I can't see where the road will lead, or how long it will be, but I have decided to follow You. Thank You for helping me when I am ill and lonely, just as You help me when I am well and brimming with happiness. This one thing I ask, Father, that You will always be with me. Amen.

Travelogue

When I die, when my spirit is freed from the limitations
    of my body,
I think I am going to fly.
I'll fly like an eagle, fly like Superman,
To wonderful places of the Earth!

I shall fly over Niagara
To hear the roar and feel the spray upon my face.
I shall fly over the great, bustling cities and the small,
    peaceful farms.
I shall fly over the Grand Canyon for one glorious,
    heart stopping sunrise.

I shall fly over the Taj Mahal to see exquisite beauty
    made by men who were created in God's image.
I shall fly over Nepal to see the great mountains
    I was too timid to climb.

I shall fly back to the morning of the Earth
And see the first man, his eyes alight with awe and
    wonder
    As he discovers his mate.

I shall fly back to see each of my children newborn,
Stroke each downy head and feel each tiny hand
Wrap tight around my finger, full of trust and promise.

Then, with a full and grateful heart,
I shall knock at the door of Heaven,
    This traveler home.

LaDonna Meinders